Understanding

GW00326603

MIGRAINE
& OTHER HEADACHES

Dr Marcia Wilkinson
& Dr Anne MacGregor

Published by Family Doctor Publications Limited
in association with the British Medical Association

© Family Doctor Publications 1999
1st edition 1993 (ISBN 1 898205 04 3)
2nd edition 1997
Reprinted 1998, 1999, 2000

Family Doctor Publications, 10 Butchers Row, Banbury, Oxon OX16 8JH

Medical Editor: Dr Tony Smith
Consultant Editor: Anne Patterson
Cover Artist: Dave Eastbury
Medical Artist: Philip Wilson & Deborah Maizels
Design: Fox Design, Godalming, Surrey
Printing: Reflex Litho, Thetford, Norfolk, using acid-free paper

ISBN: 1 898205 84 1

Contents

Common headaches

Headache is a very common symptom – over 90 per cent of the population at some time during their lives experience it, even if it is just a hangover from drinking too much alcohol. Most headaches last only a short time: a hangover headache goes after a few hours; headaches associated with an infectious illness improve when the illness is over.

These types of headache are not usually of great concern to the patient as the underlying reason is apparent.

BENIGN RECURRING HEADACHES

- Migraine

- Tension headache

- Headaches associated with pain in the muscles of the head and neck

Other headaches do not have such an obvious cause, which can lead to a great deal of concern and anxiety. Fortunately, in most cases, the headaches are not the result of anything sinister such as a brain tumour or stroke, but come under the heading of 'benign recurring headaches'.

They account for at least three-quarters of the headaches which occur and so are the commonest types of headache seen by the family doctor.

The diagnosis of these common headaches is relatively straight-forward, but depends almost entirely on the story that you tell the doctor as there is usually nothing to find on physical examination.

So how can your doctor tell which are migraines, which are tension headaches, and which are due to local muscle pains? The following accounts of some of the different headaches may give you clues about the cause of your own headaches.

MRS S'S MIGRAINE

Mrs S is a 35-year-old housewife. She is married with three children. As a child she had bilious attacks and was always car sick – so much so that her parents had to let her sit in the front seat and they always carried a bucket on long car journeys. By the time she was five, the bilious attacks were associated with mild headaches and occurred once every two or three months – often when she was excited about going to a party or to the circus.

Her periods started when she was 12. About the same time, the headaches changed – although they still only came every two to three months, the headaches were much more severe, she felt sick and could not eat, and occasionally vomited. During her late teens the headaches improved, coming only once or twice a year.

Mrs S started work as a secretary but the headaches became more frequent. She was taking the contraceptive pill and noticed that the attacks often coincided with her monthly period. At 23 she married and had her first child a year later. While pregnant with each child, she had very few attacks but they started again when she stopped breast feeding. The attacks would last for one or two days but they always seemed to come out of the blue – she could have two attacks in one month, or be free of migraine for several months.

She was 32 when she had her third child. The migraines returned but were slightly different. They started to link with her periods even though she was not on the Pill. Before the headache came on she would yawn a lot and felt tired and listless. Some attacks were preceded by bright flashes and zig-zag lines which spread across her eyes, lasting about half an hour. This was followed by the migraine she had come to know – a severe right-sided headache, feeling sick and vomiting. Often she would wake with this headache and it would last until she could get to sleep.

Mrs S went to her doctor who advised her to take an anti-sickness drug (metoclopramide) as soon as she felt an attack starting. Ten minutes later she was to take either three aspirin tablets or two paracetamol. The doctor told her to make sure that she carried at least one dose of this treatment in her handbag. She found that this simple treatment enabled her to control her attacks and she no longer had to suffer the headache for hours, lying in the dark. She is keeping a diary of her attacks to help her identify her own migraine triggers so that she can prevent the attacks starting.

Mrs J's tension headaches

Mrs J is 25 and works as a secretary for an estate agent. She has had the occasional headache, but a couple of painkillers have always been sufficient to ease the pain. Her general health has been excellent and she has seen her doctor only once in the last year, for a chest infection.

Recently, she became increasingly worried about her job. Many of her friends had been made redundant and she thought she might be next. The headaches initially came once or twice a week but then she started to wake with them every morning. They felt more like pressure round her head than an actual pain. A couple of pain killers eased them sufficiently to enable her to get to work, but the pain came back after a few hours. Getting through the day was a struggle as she found it difficult to concentrate and felt so tired. The slightest upset made her want to burst into tears. Sleep did not come easily and she often woke in the early hours, worrying about everything. Her husband is unemployed and they have difficulty keeping up with the mortgage payments on her income alone.

She went to see her doctor who prescribed a course of antidepressants. One month after starting the treatment, Mrs J's headaches improved. She had a long talk with her employer and feels more confident about her job. Her husband has found some temporary work to boost the income but long-term prospects are still uncertain. However, Mrs J is learning to take each day at a time rather than worry about things that may never happen.

Mr P's headaches due to pains in the head and neck

Mr P is 62 and is the managing director of an electronics company. When he was 30, he had a motorcycle accident but, apart from injuring his right shoulder, he did not suffer any long-term problems.

Over the past 10 years he noticed that he was having more headaches – in the last month he counted 20 days of pain. Typically the pain was worse when he woke up, or after he had done a lot of driving. Sometimes, carrying a heavy bag could trigger the pain. It was always in the same place – just behind his right ear. Sometimes he could feel it spreading from the back of the neck over his right eye. He would usually lean back in his chair and slowly circle his head as stretching his neck muscles seemed to relieve the pain. At home, he would lie in a hot bath which eased the headache. A couple of aspirin would do the trick but he was not keen on relying on painkillers.

Eventually, he got so fed up with the constant ache that he went to his general practitioner. The doctor thought that the headaches were the result of local pain in the muscles of the right shoulder and neck. Mr P has started physiotherapy and a course of anti-inflammatory drugs. His doctor has said that he may refer Mr P to a rheumatologist if the headache does not resolve with this simple treatment.

CLASSIFICATION OF HEADACHES

As you can see, each of these different headaches has specific characteristics, which are described further in *Varieties of migraine* on page 15. Although they represent the bulk of headaches seen by the family doctor, there are probably at least one hundred different causes of headache. Specialist doctors who are members of the International Headache Society have tried to classify these headaches into different groups. In addition to migraine and tension-type headache, other groups include: headaches associated with head trauma, headaches associated with vascular disorders, and headaches associated with substances or their withdrawal.

The diagnosis of these headaches depends on a combination of the patient's story, any physical signs, and the results of any tests when indicated. Some of these conditions are dealt with on pages 46–51, but is impossible and impractical to go into detail about every cause of headache in a book of this size. We hope you will find something in this book that helps you gain some understanding of your headaches and how to cope with them.

If you are in any doubt about your headaches, pay a visit to your doctor. It is much better to be reassured than to worry needlessly – especially as worry can make the headaches worse.

KEY POINTS

✓ Over 90 per cent of people have a headache at some time during their lives.

✓ Different types of headaches have different characteristics.

✓ Most headaches are not the result of anything sinister.

What is migraine?

Migraine can be defined as an episodic headache, lasting from 4 to 72 hours, associated with nausea and vomiting. Some attacks of migraine are preceded by an aura (classical migraine), typically of visual symptoms. There is complete freedom from symptoms between attacks. Daily headaches are not migraine.

The name migraine is derived from the word hemicrania meaning a one-sided headache, although the headache can be generalized. But migraine is more than just a headache and the headache is not necessarily the major symptom. Most people feel sick and are often unable to continue their normal daily activities.

Some have to lie still in a quiet, darkened room until the attack is over. Many cannot bear even the thought of food but others find eating takes the edge off the nausea.

SYMPTOMS OF MIGRAINE

- Headache
- Visual disturbances
- Feeling sick
- Vomiting
- Aversion to light
- Aversion to food
- Lethargy

Migraine has been likened to a power cut as the whole body seems to shut down until the attack is over. Lethargy is a common symptom and every task seems to take twice as long – if it is possible to tackle it at all. The stomach stops functioning normally, making it harder for medication to be absorbed into the bloodstream, especially if treatment is delayed. Sometimes an attack ends with vomiting but in most cases the headache improves after a good sleep or gradually fades away.

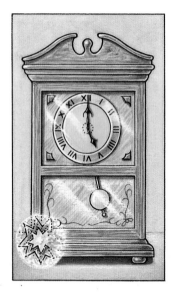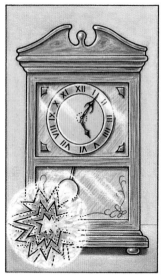

Visual distortion in a migraine aura.

An attack of migraine can be very frightening. Those experiencing the visual disturbances of the aura are often scared of permanently losing their vision. Strokes and brain tumours are also common fears. Fortunately, such sinister causes are rare and other symptoms may be apparent before headaches. Although the symptoms of migraine can be disturbing, they are not life threatening and the body returns to normal between attacks.

DURATION OF ATTACKS

The headache of a migraine usually eases within 24 hours of starting but can last anything from part of a day to three days. Often it takes another day or so to get back to normal as symptoms of tiredness and feeling washed out remain even after the headache has gone. A few feel extra well after an attack – possibly due to relief that the attack is over.

Children often have short and sharp attacks lasting only a few hours. With increasing age the attacks typically last longer but are less severe, and the aura may become more frequent.

Between attacks sufferers feel their usual selves – forgetting how bad they felt until the next attack.

FREQUENCY OF ATTACKS

The frequency of migraine varies considerably both between individuals and in the same person. The attacks may come once or twice a month during a bad patch but a few unlucky people might have a spell of attacks occurring once or twice a week. This could be followed by a gap of several months or even years without an attack, for no apparent reason. In general, attacks become less frequent after the age of 55 although this is not always the case.

HOW COMMON IS MIGRAINE?

At a conservative estimate, migraine affects at least five million people in the UK, i.e. about 10 per cent of the population. It is difficult to give a precise figure because some people may only have three or four attacks in a lifetime and not recognize them as migraines. Most population studies to date are based on the results of questionnaires. These can give misleading figures as it is very difficult to diagnose migraine correctly by questionnaire.

Although migraine affects at least 10 per cent of the population, it is difficult to assess how common the condition is and how many new cases there are, partly because so few people with migraine visit the doctor.

Many sufferers have seen close relatives struggle through attacks and are under the false impression that little can be done to help them.

Others feel they are wasting the doctor's time because between attacks they are healthy.

Another problem is that a universally accepted definition of migraine was only introduced in 1988. Previous studies undertaken before this date used inconsistent criteria, therefore making it impossible to compare results.

However, several studies have been undertaken using the new definition and the results from different countries are similar.

In Denmark, 1,000 men and women aged between 25 and 64 were interviewed about their general health and headaches. The researchers found that eight per cent of men and 25 per cent of women questioned had had an attack of migraine at some time in their lives.

A survey in America set out to analyse the results of a questionnaire sent to 15,000 households. Replies were received from 63 per cent of people aged between 12 and 80. From this group, six per cent of men and 18 per cent of women reported having one or more migraine headaches each year.

WHO GETS MIGRAINE?
Sex

Migraine affects more women than men – the ratio is three to one. Hormonal changes in women are the obvious reason for this difference between the sexes and accounts for the fact that, until puberty, migraine is equally prevalent in boys and girls.

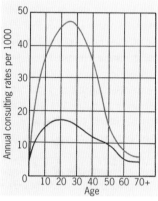

Differences in the consulting rates of males and females according to age.

Age

At least 90 per cent of the population with migraine have their first attack before the age of 40. For most people the migraine starts during their teens or early twenties, although it has been diagnosed in young children and even babies. It is rare for migraine to start in people over the age of 50.

Even though migraine starts in the young, it may not become a problem until later life. Studies show that women are most likely to have problems with migraine when they reach middle age. In men the pattern is fairly consistent throughout their lives.

Migraine usually improves in later life for both sexes, although a few continue to have attacks.

Intelligence

For many years it was thought that migraine sufferers were more intelligent than non-sufferers. This myth was dispelled when it was found that people who have had more years of education are more likely to seek treatment from a doctor. In fact migraine affects people from all walks of life regardless of race, intelligence or social class.

TRIGGER FACTORS

Although doctors do not know why people get migraine, it is known that certain factors are involved in triggering an attack. Most people have read or been told that they should avoid cheese, chocolate and red wine if they have migraine.

Unfortunately, for most people simply avoiding certain foods is insufficient to prevent the attacks. This is because trigger factors build up over a period of time and act in combination to cross the threshold of an attack. This explains why missing a meal or having a glass of wine does not always trigger an attack.

If you drink a glass of wine when other triggers are present, such as after an exhausting and stressful day at work or around the time of your period, an attack may result.

Triggers may change over the years even though the attacks themselves are the same. Stress, late nights etc. may have been the most important triggers when you were younger but in later years neck and back problems may play a greater role.

Specific foods

Twenty per cent of sufferers link certain foods to their migraine. The most common foods are chocolate, cheese and citrus fruits, commonly referred to as the three Cs. Alcohol, particularly red wine, is also a recognized trigger.

There is clear evidence that certain foods can provoke migraine in a few susceptible individuals. There is no scientific evidence that migraine has an allergic basis and food intolerance is a more accepted term.

Allergy tests are of little value in testing for intolerance to implicated foods as the tests are not sensitive or specific enough.

TRIGGER FACTORS OF MIGRAINE ATTACKS

INSUFFICIENT FOOD
- Missing meals
- Delayed meals
- Inadequate quantity

SPECIFIC FOODS
- Cheese, chocolate, citrus fruits
- Alcohol
- Coffee, tea
- Sweet snacks

SLEEP
- Lying in
- Lack of sleep

HEAD AND NECK PAINS
- Eyes, sinuses, neck, teeth or jaw pain

EMOTIONAL TRIGGERS

ENVIRONMENTAL TRIGGERS
- Bright or flickering lights
- Over-exertion
- Travel
- Weather changes
- Strong smells

HORMONAL FACTORS (WOMEN)
- Pregnancy
- Oral contraception
- HRT
- Menstruation

Not all the above apply to every migraine patient and usually more than one factor has to be present to initiate an attack.

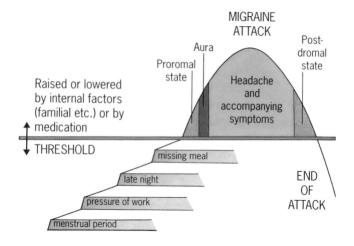

MIGRAINE ATTACK

Aura

Proromal state

Post-dromal state

Headache and accompanying symptoms

Raised or lowered by internal factors (familial etc.) or by medication

THRESHOLD

missing meal

late night

pressure of work

menstrual period

END OF ATTACK

Diagram illustrating the idea of the need for several precipitating factors acting in combination to cross the 'threshold' of initiation of an attack of migraine. The prodromal state is the name given to early warning symptoms.

Whatever the mechanism, many people strictly avoid suspect foods without first discovering whether or not they contribute to their own headache. Anyone who thinks that a certain food is precipitating attacks should eliminate that food from their diet for two months, keeping a diary to see if there is any change in their attacks. If the frequency of attacks is unchanged, the food can be reinstated and another suspected food eliminated for a further two months. However, the only certain way of identifying food triggers is to avoid all suspected foods by following a strict elimination diet. This should only be done under the supervision of a doctor or dietician because of the risk of malnutrition.

Most people find that they can control their migraines by identifying other triggers, making only minimal changes to their diet.

Lack of food

Missing meals, snack lunches or eating sugary snacks instead of a proper meal can all lead to an attack. Breakfast is a particularly important meal. Some migraine sufferers have controlled their attacks by eating small nutritious snacks at frequent intervals.

Changes in sleeping pattern

Sleepless nights, overwork and too many late nights can result in becoming over-tired and triggering a migraine. Conversely, sleeping in, even for just half-an-hour longer than usual or lying in bed dozing, starts up a headache in many people. Unfortunately, this is often at a weekend when they want to relax.

Hormonal changes in women
Many women relate their attacks to the menstrual cycle and may have had their first migraine around the time of their first period. Taking the oral contraceptive pill can aggravate migraine, although a few women do notice an improvement.

It is wise to stop the Pill if attacks become more frequent or more severe. It should not be taken by women who have attacks of classical migraine and should be discontinued by those whose attacks convert from common to classical.

Pregnancy usually leads to an improvement in migraine after the first trimester but attacks return after the baby is born.

The menopause is the most difficult time for women with migraine but little is known about the effects of hormone replacement therapy on migraine in women. The link between headaches and hormones is covered in pages 27–32.

Head and neck pain
Muscle tension affecting the neck and shoulder muscles is a common problem, particularly if you sit hunched over a desk or VDU all day or do a lot of driving. Local pain in the head and neck can cause headaches as well as triggering migraine.

As your body ages the bones undergo arthritic changes which sometimes aggravate migraine because this puts the muscles that support the bones under more stress.

In a few cases, migraine can be aggravated by specific dental problems such as problems with wisdom teeth, bite and jaw joint. It is worthwhile checking with your dentist, especially if you grind your teeth at night or have problems with your jaw locking when you open your mouth wide.

Exercise
Hard physical exercise, especially if you are unfit, can be a trigger. Regular exercise, without overdoing it, can help prevent migraine attacks. It can help breathing and strengthen muscles.

Exercise also stimulates the body to release its own natural pain killers and promotes a general sense of well-being.

Travel
Be careful on long journeys, especially if they involve a change in meal and sleep patterns. Allow enough time so that you are not rushed, and take something to eat in case meals are delayed.

Stress

Anxiety and emotion do play an important part in migraine but other triggers such as missing meals or not sleeping properly often go hand in hand with stress. Some people have more attacks when under stress; others cope with stress but have attacks when they eventually have a chance to relax. Even pleasant things can be stressful, for example, promotion at work or a heavy, but interesting, assignment. Stress in one guise or another is unavoidable but it is important to recognize that these stresses exist and find ways of dealing with at least some of them.

Other causes

Bright lights, loud noise, strong smells, changes in the weather, smoky environments and hot stuffy rooms (such as the cinema) can all trigger attacks in susceptible people. Why do some people get migraine and not others? Pain is usually nature's way of telling you that something is wrong and helps to prevent further injury to the body, so an attack of migraine may have a protective role against a build up of triggers. It is generally thought that migraine can run in families, typically from mother to daughter. Although it is true to say that migraine sufferers usually have a family history of migraine, no specific gene has been identified.

Migraine is such a common condition that there is a high likelihood of there being at least one other member of the family with migraine without it being an inherited condition but researchers continue to look for a genetic link. It is possible that everyone has the potential to experience migraine but that the threshold for an attack is higher in some people than in others.

These people would need a greater number of triggers present at any one time to precipitate an attack than those people with a lower threshold.

KEY POINTS

✓ Migraine is an episodic headache, lasting four to 72 hours, associated with nausea and vomiting.

✓ The frequency of attacks varies between individuals and in the same person.

✓ Migraine affects women more than men and rarely starts after the age of 50.

✓ Changes in blood flow to the brain are thought to underlie migraine attacks but trigger factors are also involved.

What causes migraine?

The many symptoms of migraine have led to a variety of ideas as to the cause. Aretaeus of Cappadocia (early second century AD) attributed the condition to cold and dry weather. Galen thought that it was caused by irritation of the brain by black bile. Serapion, in the ninth century, attributed the condition to hot or cold substances in the digestive tract being transported to the brain.

It was not until the seventeenth century that more scientific arguments were considered. Thomas Willis was aware of many of the triggers for migraine, including diet. He also speculated that the headache of migraine could result from expansion of the blood vessels in the head.

THE VASCULAR THEORY

This vascular theory has remained to the present day and, indeed, many of the treatments used for migraine are believed to act by constricting the swollen vessels. In the late eighteenth century, Erasmus Darwin (grandfather of Charles Darwin) suggested that spinning a patient around in a centrifuge would force blood from the head to the feet and relieve the swelling. Fortunately, such treatment was not practised.

NEUROLOGICAL THEORIES

In 1873, Edward Liveing theorized that migraine was caused by nerve storms, or discharges, originating in the brain. Other researchers have followed with similar neurological arguments. This has led to continuing, sometimes heated, debate as to which of the two theories – the neurological or the vascular – is correct.

Doctors now agree that both aspects are important. Certainly, alterations in the size of the blood vessels do seem to account for at least some of the features of an attack but these events appear to be initiated by other changes within the nervous system.

NEUROTRANSMITTERS

More recently, scientists have studied the role of certain chemical messengers within the brain called neurotransmitters. Research has strongly implicated the role of serotonin (also called 5-hydroxy-tryptamine, or 5HT). Measurable changes in the concentration of this chemical occur during a migraine attack as it is released from its storage sites within the body. It was found that an injection of serotonin could effectively abort an attack. Unfortunately, serotonin cannot be used as a treatment because it causes many unacceptable side effects.

However, many of the drugs used in the treatment of migraine have some action on the serotonin pathways in the brain (see page 39).

KEY POINTS

✓ According to one theory the headache of migraine results from expansion of blood vessels in the head.

✓ The neurological theory holds that it has a neurological basis – changes within the nervous system.

✓ Certain chemical messengers in the brain, called neurotransmitters, have recently been implicated, notably 5-hydroxytryptamine or serotonin.

✓ Many of the drugs used in migraine treatment have some action on serotonin.

Varieties of migraine

About 10 per cent of the population in the United Kingdom have migraine and regular sufferers describe it as the worst headache in the world.

There are two main types of migraine: classical migraine, called migraine with aura in the International Headache Classification, and common migraine, also known as migraine without aura. It is possible to have both types of migraine: 70 per cent of people who have attacks of classical migraine also have attacks of common migraine. These are usually the same as their classical attacks, but without the aura. About one per cent of migraine sufferers have attacks of the aura alone, with no subsequent headache.

In both types of migraine, the headaches are usually on one side of the head but may occasionally be on both sides. One of the unusual characteristics of the headache is that the side may vary and although, for instance, one sufferer usually has attacks affecting the right side of the head, in some attacks it may affect the left side. The pain varies greatly in severity, ranging from a dull nagging ache to an unbearable pounding.

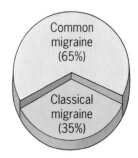

Common migraine (65%)

Classical migraine (35%)

There are two main types of migraine.

As well as the headache most people feel sick and about 25 per cent actually vomit. A few people also suffer from diarrhoea.

A migraine attack lasts from a few hours to 72 hours and there is a period free of symptoms of at least 72 hours – usually longer – between attacks.

A continuous daily headache is never due to migraine.

CLASSICAL MIGRAINE

This is the most dramatic form of migraine, but constitutes only about 35 per cent of all migraine attacks. The headache, nausea and vomiting are preceded by flashing lights or other sensory symptoms. The migraine attack itself consists of four phases: the prodromal state (early warning symptoms), the aura, the headache and recovery.

Prodromes

Most people do not at first recognize the prodromal state because the symptoms are indefinite. They include:

● tiredness
● yawning
● increased awareness of what is happening
● overactivity
● fluid retention
● craving for food – particularly sweet things such as chocolate.

Sometimes these symptoms are recognized by other members of the family and only later by the sufferer.

These symptoms can last from an hour or two, up to 24 hours.

Aura

The next phase is the aura, which lasts from 10 to 60 minutes. The term aura has been used to describe the symptoms preceding a migraine attack. These include:

● disturbances of vision
● speech disorders
● weakness
● sensory disorders.

A remarkable variety of visual disturbances may be experienced during the aura. The simplest consists of brilliant stars, sparks, flashes, zig-zags, or simple geometric patterns which pass across the visual field. A sufferer may complain of bright stars in front of the eyes, sometimes with one star brighter than the rest, starting from the lower corner of the visual field and passing rapidly across it. At other times the aura consists of rippling, shimmering or undulations in the visual field, or even a temporary loss of sight in one part of the field. Zig-zagging lights resembling a fortified castle (called fortification spectra) may also occur.

Sensory symptoms include tingling and pins and needles, which are usually in one or other hand or arm, or around the mouth. The tingling sensation typically starts in the fingers and gradually spreads up the arms over a period of 15–20 minutes.

Sometimes there is difficulty in speaking, mental confusion, or weakness of the arm, but these do not occur often.

These symptoms recede after 10 to 60 minutes, and are followed by headache, nausea, and vomiting. If any of these symptoms persist for more than an hour, you should go and see your doctor as they may be caused by some more serious underlying condition.

Other features

● **Headache:** The headache is typically one-sided and may be very severe. In about one-third of patients it is bilateral. It lasts from 4 to 72 hours. The pain is usually in the forehead or temples but may start from the back of the neck. It often starts in the early morning so that the patient wakes up with the pain.

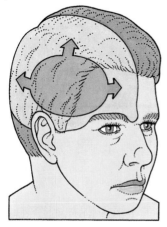

Distribution of pain in migraine.

● **Photophobia:** Dislike of light, photophobia, occurs in about 80 per cent of attacks, and is found in both common as well as classical migraine.

● **Nausea:** Nausea occurs in about 95 per cent of the attacks, vomiting in about 25 per cent, and diarrhoea in 20 per cent. Sometimes the vomiting is so severe that the sufferer cannot take tablets. If this is the case, the treatment must be taken as a suppository, by inhaler or by injection.

COMMON MIGRAINE

In this type of migraine the attack is similar to that of the classical migraine attack, starting with the prodromal stage, but there is no aura. As its name suggests, common migraine is the commonest form and accounts for about 65 per cent of migraine attacks.

Cluster headache

This is usually considered to be a part of the migraine syndrome but it differs from classical and common migraine in many respects.

It occurs in men, rather than women, and affects an older age group. About four per cent of migraine sufferers have this type of headache.

Cluster headache is so called because of its tendency to occur in bouts, each of which lasts from four to eight weeks.

The attack builds up within a few minutes, lasting about 45 minutes in total. Several attacks may occur each day during the cluster period, typically waking the sufferer from his or her sleep.

The pain always affects the same side of the head in each bout and is felt as a severe pain and around the eye. It may radiate above the eye to the temple, jaw or gums, on the same side of or, more rarely, over half the head. When the pain is bad, the pupil on the affected side may constrict, the eye reddens and waters, and occasionally the eyelid droops.

Some patients sweat excessively, particularly on the affected side of the face. The nostril may seem to be blocked and the skin on that side may be hypersensitive.

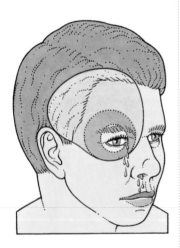

Distribution of pain in a cluster headache.

The pain of cluster headaches is so severe and distressing that the sufferer often paces up and down, or rocks back and forth, trying to find ways to distract himself from the agony.

This excruciating pain can be pulsating or throbbing but it is usually described as burning, boring, piercing, tearing or grinding. During a bout and between the attacks, the area around the eye can feel bruised.

Many sufferers can bring on attacks by drinking alcohol during a bout, although they are able to drink when they are out of the cluster period.

OTHER VARIETIES OF MIGRAINE

There are other less common varieties of migraine. One rare type is ophthalmoplegic migraine. This occurs in young people aged 6–12 and, in addition to the headache, there may be weakness of one of the eye muscles. In another type which doctors call basilar migraine, dizziness, unsteadiness, or difficulty in talking may be associated with the headache. Another very rare type is hemiplegic migraine. In this there is a recurrent weakness of one side of the body. Very often there is a history of similar attacks in another member of the family, and the weakness is usually on the same side.

KEY POINTS

✓ There are two main types of migraine – classical migraine (35 per cent of attacks) and common migraine (65 per cent of attacks).

✓ The migraine attack consists of four phases: the prodromal state, the aura, the headache and recovery.

✓ The pain of migraine is usually in the forehead or temples. It is usually one-sided and can be very severe.

✓ The pain of cluster headache (considered to be part of the migraine syndrome) is felt in and around the eye, sometimes radiating to the temple, jaw or gums on the same side.

Diagnosis of migraine

Migraine is difficult to diagnose because there are no specific tests for it – the diagnosis depends on the history and examination. Questions about the frequency, type, site of the headache, and the trigger factors, help to make the diagnosis. Migraine, tension headache and localized muscle pain together make up 90 per cent of headaches referred by family doctors for a consultant opinion. Diagnosis is comparatively easy when these headaches occur separately but when two or more occur together, as they frequently do, it is much more difficult.

Before the rare types are diagnosed, all other possible diagnoses must be excluded. This may mean being referred by your family doctor to a neurologist who will take a careful history and examine you, as well as possibly doing a CT (computed tomography) or MRI (magnetic resonance imaging) scan. These are specialized but quite painless ways of visualizing the brain and skull.

However, these tests are very expensive so they are only done when the neurologist thinks they are essential.

KEY POINTS

✓ There are no specific tests – diagnosis depends on the history and examination of the sufferer.

How to live with migraine

Many people hide the fact that they have migraine from friends, family and people at work, often afraid that they will be labelled as neurotic. This is a myth that doctors and health workers are trying to dispel, in order to help both sufferers and non-sufferers realize that migraine is an organic condition, and that it should be treated seriously.

The Migraine Action Association is a self-help organization run by sufferers for sufferers. At a recent meeting members were asked if they considered that there is a social stigma associated with migraine. Nearly three-quarters of the audience replied 'yes'. Two-thirds also said that they continued to soldier on during an attack because they did not feel that others took migraine seriously. Some were afraid of losing their jobs if they took time off from work because of what their boss saw as just a headache.

Those at home are no better off: trying to cope with boisterous children and running a house while in the throes of an attack is very difficult.

Migraine can disrupt the life of the sufferer, who appears completely well to all those who have never seen the person during an attack. This makes it harder for non-sufferers to realize the extent of the problem.

Most sufferers manage to struggle on through the rest of the day at work or at home but collapse into bed as soon as they can. Social engagements have to be cancelled and family life is disrupted, affecting relationships with close family and friends. Work may not be seriously affected but leisure time is lost.

The extent of the problem obviously depends on the severity of the symptoms as well as the frequency and duration of attacks. Fortunately, most migraine sufferers have infrequent attacks and manage to cope with the help of painkillers. It is only when attacks worsen or become more frequent that they seek help from a doctor. Studies show that 70 per cent cope alone, only 30 per cent visiting their GP.

This is an unfortunate situation as, although there is no cure for migraine, there are numerous ways of controlling migraine both with and without the use of drugs. Finding ways of managing migraine is not always easy but you are much more likely to succeed if you can enrol the help of family and friends and obtain advice from your GP or a specialist centre.

Migraine is an individual problem and your best line of management will probably be different from that of other migraine sufferers you know. Try simple things first, one at a time. If you do not feel you are getting anywhere, speak to your GP. You can always ask to be referred to a specialist migraine clinic – see the list of Useful addresses on page 57.

SELF-HELP PREVENTION
Keep an attack diary
It is important to keep an accurate record of your attacks to help you try to establish any patterns. Fortunately, the body is good at forgetting pain which is why whenever you have an attack you say that you must do something about the migraine, yet between attacks you forget ... until the next time. Keeping the record means that you have documented evidence of each attack that you can analyse.

Keep a trigger diary
Trigger diaries can help you unravel the mystery of why you get attacks. Triggers (discussed in more detail on page 9) usually act in combination, building up to a threshold, and triggering the attack. A few people are aware of at least some of their triggers. Others are confused when a suspect trigger sometimes results in an attack, but not every time.

Rather than 'What triggers an attack?' a more useful question is 'How many triggers do you need to initiate an attack?' Even your usual daily routine can include triggers of which you are not aware because you remain below the threshold of an attack until a few extra triggers crop up. It is important to keep a record of potential triggers every day as you are unlikely to remember them clearly when you are having an attack.

Look at the list of common triggers every day, just before you go to bed. Make a note of any that you suspect were present that day, such as shopping or a delayed meal, etc. Women should keep a record of their menstrual period and any premenstrual symptoms. If you take any regular medication, including vitamins or tablets from the health food shop, make a note of these. Similarly, record if you take the oral contraceptive pill or HRT.

	Jan	Apr	Sep	Oct	Nov
1					
2					
3					
4					
5					
6					
7					
8					
9					\
10					⊘
11			⊗		O
12			O		O
13	\		X	O	O
14	\	\	⊗	O	O
15	X	⊗	O	O	
16	X	O	O		
17	O	O	O		
18	O	O	O		
19	O	O			
20	O				
21	O				
22					
23					
24					
25					
26					
27					
28					
29					
30					
31					

X migraine

\ non-migraine headache

O menstrual bleed

Record of a patient with 'menstrual migraine'. A similar chart for a patient on the oral contraceptive pill might show attacks occurring during the withdrawal bleed of the pill-free week.

Identifying triggers

You should continue to complete the trigger diary and the attack diary until you have had at least five attacks. Compare the information in each and see if there was a build up of triggers coinciding with the attacks. Looking back on the attacks, were there any warning signs?

Study the list of triggers and you should be able to divide them into two groups – those that you can do something about (e.g. missing meals, drinking red wine) and those that are out of your control (e.g. menstrual cycle, travelling). First, try to deal with the triggers over which you have some influence. Cut out suspect triggers one at a time – if you try to deal with them all at once you will not know which are most relevant to you. Try to compensate so that, if you are having a particularly stressful time, you take care to eat regularly and find ways to unwind before you go to bed.

If your attacks regularly start late morning or late afternoon, look at your meal times. A mid-morning or mid-afternoon snack may be all that is necessary to prevent the attacks. Similarly, if you have an early evening meal and wake with an attack, try a snack before you go to bed.

Certain foods, in particular cheese, chocolate, alcohol, citrus fruits, dairy produce and many others have been implicated in triggering migraine. Because several factors are necessary to trigger an attack it follows that, if other factors can be identified and minimized, food triggers will be less important.

If you do suspect that any foods trigger an attack, cut them out of your diet for a few weeks before re-introducing them.

You may need to do this with the same food more than once as a check. If you think a large number of foods is involved, visit your doctor, as elimination diets run the risk of causing malnutrition if they are not adequately supervised.

SELF-HELP TREATMENT
Identify prodromal symptoms
Prodromes are the warning symptoms that precede the headache by several hours, sometimes the evening or day before. These subtle changes in mood or behaviour can be present before attacks of classical or common migraine. The symptoms may go unnoticed until attention is drawn to them and are often more apparent to friends and relatives than to the sufferer. Clumsiness, yawning and feeling tired and irritable are common prodromes. Others include a stiff neck, feeling thirsty, and sensitivity to light and sound.

Some prodromal symptoms get incorrectly blamed as triggers for the attack. A craving for sweet foods may result in a desire to eat chocolate or other sweet foods. A few people feel on top of the world before an attack and rush around, thinking later that the attack was caused by over-activity. These are signs that the attack has already begun.

Recognition of these prodromal symptoms can be of enormous benefit as avoiding known trigger factors during this time may be all that is necessary to stop the attack developing further.

Always carry at least a single dose of your preferred medication so that you can take it as soon as you feel an attack coming on. It is important to take medication early, as it is more likely to be effective. The stomach is less active during a migraine so that drugs taken by mouth are not absorbed into the blood stream as well as they would be normally.

What to do during an attack

Try to eat something if you can. Bland food, such as dry toast or a biscuit, can ease the nausea. If you do vomit, it is much less painful if you have eaten something than retching on an empty stomach. Some people prefer to eat something sweet; others prefer to have a fizzy drink such as lemonade, or a cup of tea with sugar.

In an ideal world you should give in to the attack and try to rest. Sleep is nature's way of aiding recovery, and struggling on through the migraine usually only prolongs the attack. Obviously not everyone can pack up work and go to bed but at least try to take things more slowly.

Catch up on more menial tasks rather than doing something that requires concentration. Eat small, frequent snacks and take painkillers to keep the attack at bay.

Try putting a covered hot water bottle or an ice pack on the back of your neck or on the most painful point. Cover your eyes with a mask – you can buy one from the chemist. Although many prefer to lie in bed, a few find it more comfortable to sit propped up in a chair.

Do whatever seems natural to minimize the pain.

WHEN TO SEE A DOCTOR

If you feel that you can manage your migraines yourself, there is no need to see your doctor. If there is any doubt about the cause of your headaches, or if the pattern of your headaches changes, it is important to visit your doctor to make sure of the correct diagnosis.

Very few headaches are due to anything serious but they can sometimes be a symptom of an underlying medical problem.

Do not think that you are wasting the doctor's time. It is much better to be reassured than to worry that there is something wrong.

A great deal can be done to help headaches without the need for drugs.

Otherwise, your GP can advise on the correct use of tablets from the pharmacy or there are drugs which can be prescribed for migraine.

Even if you have seen your doctor in the past with little success, it is worth going again as you may need to try more than one type of treatment before you find the one that suits you best.

Take your trigger and attack diaries with you. List the various treatments you have already tried, how you took them, and what effect they had. Make a note of when your headaches first started and how they have changed over the years. This information will help your doctor to assess the problem more quickly and make it easier to tailor the treatment to your individual needs. Because there are no tests for migraine, your doctor cannot tell if the treatment he suggests first is going to be the most effective so be prepared for several visits. There is no cure for migraine but treatment can help you regain control over the attacks.

KEY POINTS

✓ To help establish any patterns, keep an accurate record of your attacks and what seems to trigger them.

✓ Cut out suspect triggers one at a time.

✓ Try to rest during an attack.

✓ Do not cut out a large number of foods without visiting your doctor first.

✓ Do not be afraid to visit your doctor if you are worried.

Headaches in women

You do not have to be an expert to realize that women suffer more headaches than men: 'Not tonight dear, I've got a headache', is a popular joke.

The link between migraine and menstruation was first recorded by Hippocrates in the fifth century BC. For many centuries doctors believed that the womb was the source of the headaches. Doctors now realize that the mechanism of hormonal headaches is much more complex. An organ in the brain, the hypothalamus, operates a complex control system of the menstrual cycle, sending messages to the ovaries and the uterus. It seems more likely that hormonal headaches are initiated within the brain than by the uterus or ovaries.

HEADACHES AND HORMONES

Few studies have looked at the effect of hormones on non-migraine headaches but studies of women attending the City of London Migraine Clinic show that women are more prone to non-migraine headaches around the time of their period, even if they also suffer from migraine. Headaches are also a recognized symptom of the pre-menstrual syndrome and of the menopause. Some women notice more headaches when they start the oral contraceptive pill. These usually settle after a few months but occasionally it is necessary to change to a different type of contraceptive pill. Apart from these specific events, hormonal changes have little effect on non-migraine headaches.

MENSTRUAL MIGRAINE

In another study undertaken at the City of London Migraine Clinic, 50 per cent of women thought that their migraine attacks were linked to their menstrual cycle. Of the women questioned 15 per cent reported that they had their first attack of migraine in the same year as their first period. Further studies show that these initial attacks are often irregular, occurring at any time of the cycle, but by the time a woman reaches her mid to late thirties, she may notice that the attacks establish a monthly pattern. Sometimes this pattern only becomes apparent when the periods return after the birth of a baby.

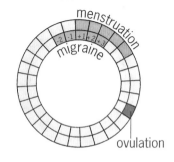

Relationship between migraine and the menstrual cycle.

As the result of our research, we found that about 10 per cent of women regularly had attacks of migraine within the two days before their period started and the first three days of bleeding (days −2 to +3) and at no other time of the month. We defined this as 'menstrual migraine'.

Menstrual migraine has been linked to the drop in oestrogen that naturally occurs during the menstrual cycle. There is no need to do any tests to check the hormones in these women as there is nothing wrong; it seems that women with menstrual migraine are just more sensitive to normal hormonal fluctuations.

Although it is possible to use oestrogen supplements to prevent the drop in oestrogen, studies show that such treatment is not effective for every woman with menstrual migraine. Research is being directed at other chemicals that change with the menstrual cycle, such as prostaglandins, which may also play a part.

Non-hormonal triggers for migraine are also important in menstrual migraine. Studies show that the changing levels of hormones also affect other migraine triggers; for example, women are more susceptible to the effects of alcohol and missing meals around the time of their period.

SELF-HELP

If you suspect a link between your periods and attacks of migraine, the first thing to do is keep a diary. This helps to establish the exact relationship of the timing of attacks and the different stages of the cycle. Keep a note of any premenstrual symptoms such as craving for sweet foods, breast tenderness, etc., as well as an accurate record of the migraine attacks and menstrual periods. For each attack, jot down the time it started, how long it lasted, and what symptoms you experienced. Also keep a note of what treatment you took, what time you took it, and how effective it was. Mention if the period was unusually painful or heavy. Also keep a note of any non-hormonal triggers that could have been responsible (see page 9).

After a few months, look back over the records and see if you can establish any patterns. Look especially at the non-hormonal migraine triggers, as avoiding these premenstrually may be sufficient to prevent what appears to be an hormonally linked attack; i.e. take care not to get over-tired and, if necessary, cut out alcohol and eat small, frequent snacks to keep blood sugar levels up as missing meals or going too long without food can trigger attacks.

Treating other premenstrual symptoms can also help and it may be worth trying supplements of vitamin B_6 or evening primrose oil, which are available from the chemist.

See your doctor for advice if you have severe symptoms, or if the attacks remain unchanged after trying these simple methods for a few months.

ORAL CONTRACEPTION

Most women with migraine who take the combined oral contra-ceptive pill – the Pill – do not notice any change in their attacks. A few even notice an improvement but the attacks may become more severe or frequent, typically during the Pill-free week at the time of the monthly 'period'.

Non-migraine headaches are also more common. Many of these problems settle down eventually so it is worthwhile continuing with the Pill for a few months before stopping.

Most doctors feel that it is safe for women with migraine to take the Pill unless they have classical migraine with an aura. Sometimes a woman with common migraine experiences attacks with an aura when she starts the Pill. In these cases the Pill should be stopped and an alternative form of contraception used.

These guidelines are based on studies of the early Pill, when it was feared that women with migraine were more susceptible to some of its unwanted effects. The original Pill contained high doses of oestro-gen which affected blood clotting and increased the risk of thrombosis in all women, whether or not they had migraine, but particularly smokers.

The modern Pill contains much lower doses of oestrogen and the overall risk of thrombosis is very low in healthy women under the age of 40 who do not smoke.

It therefore seems unlikely that the Pill has any great impact on migraine nowadays but it is wise to err on the side of caution. Women who wish to continue with oral contraception can take the progesterone-only mini-Pill which has minimal effect on clotting.

PREGNANCY

It is often stated that migraine improves during pregnancy but, in reality, this is not always so. One study showed that 64 per cent of women had fewer or less severe attacks if their migraine had previously been linked to menstruation; only 48 per cent of women noticed an improvement when pregnant.

In general, migraine may be more severe in the early weeks of pregnancy but, after three months, about 70 per cent of women notice an improvement. In the remaining women, migraine remains unchanged or worsens. Occasionally, women may have their first attack of migraine when pregnant or start to have attacks with an aura which they did not have before.

Some women have an attack within a few hours of giving birth. After childbirth, attacks can result from interrupted sleep or an increase of other migraine triggers. It is not uncommon for attacks to return when the periods restart – often becoming more closely linked to the menstrual cycle – although for most women the migraine eventually reverts to its former type and frequency.

Treating migraine in pregnancy can be difficult because of the restriction on taking medication. Paracetamol is safe and should be taken as soon as an attack starts. Eat small frequent meals to prevent drops in blood sugar and make sure that you take adequate rest. There is no point struggling on through a migraine, particularly when you are pregnant, as it only delays the inevitable.

Follow the self-help suggestions on pages 24–25 and speak to your doctor or obstetrician for further advice.

HYSTERECTOMY

There is no evidence to suggest that a hysterectomy is of any benefit in the treatment of hormonal headaches. The normal menstrual cycle is the result of the interaction of several different organs in the body. These include organs in the brain, in addition to the ovaries and the uterus.

Removing the uterus alone has little effect on the hormonal fluctuations of the menstrual cycle even though the periods cease.

THE MENOPAUSE

The largest group of people who visit the City of London Migraine

Clinic for advice are women in their early forties. In the years leading up to a woman's final period, the menopause, the ovaries produce diminishing amounts of oestrogen. During this time of hormonal imbalance, it is not unusual for migraine attacks to become more frequent or severe.

The few studies that have been undertaken suggest that the menopause aggravates migraine in up to 45 per cent of women; between 30 and 45 per cent do not notice any change and about 15 per cent notice an improvement. At least some of the increase in headaches around the menopause is not directly caused by hormones: women experiencing frequent night sweats may lose sleep – over-tiredness is itself a migraine trigger.

For most women migraine settles after the menopause. This is possibly because the hormonal fluctuations cease and the concentration of oestrogen stabilizes at lower levels. A few women continue to have attacks which can sometimes follow a cyclical pattern years after the menopause. The reason for this is unclear.

HORMONE REPLACEMENT THERAPY (HRT)

HRT was introduced as a means of replacing the oestrogen which the ovaries stop producing after the menopause. Initially it was used as a treatment for hot flushes, night sweats and other menopausal symptoms. The natural oestrogens used for HRT have quite different effects from the potent synthetic oestrogens used in the Pill and protect against, rather than increase, the risk of thrombosis. Recently, studies suggest that if HRT is taken for several years, it can reduce the risk of heart disease, strokes and fractures.

But HRT is neither suitable nor necessary for every woman, and it is not without problems. Unless a woman has had a hysterectomy, she must take regular courses of progestogen, which recreates a monthly period. This is similar to the hormone progesterone that a woman naturally produces during the menstrual cycle.

Progestogen is necessary to prevent the oestrogen over-stimulating the lining of the womb, which can lead to cancerous changes.

Several researchers have noticed that women report more headaches during, or shortly after, the course of progestogen, in addition to other symptoms which are very similar to those reported in the premenstrual syndrome – tender breasts, fluid retention, irritability and depression.

Very few studies have assessed the effect of HRT on migraine, a problem compounded by the vast number of different types and methods of HRT available – daily pills or gel, patches changed once or twice a week, or implants inserted under the skin every six months. Like all hormonal events, HRT may aggravate migraine in some women but lead to an improvement in others. The only way to find out is to try it. Whichever type of HRT you start with, it is important to give it an adequate trial; the first three months is a time of imbalance as the body becomes accustomed to the change of hormones. If you are unhappy with one type of HRT, it is worth switching to a different type or trying a different route. Keep a record of all headaches, both migraine and non-migraine, before and during treatment.

KEY POINTS

✓ Fifty per cent of women in one study thought that their migraine attacks were linked to their menstrual cycle.

✓ It is unlikely that the Pill has any great impact on migraine.

✓ HRT may aggravate migraine in some postmenopausal women but lead to an improvement in others. The only way to find out is to try it.

✓ If you suspect a link between your periods and attacks of migraine, keep a diary.

Headaches in children

Children, as well as adults, have headaches. These are sometimes difficult to diagnose in the under-fives but even at this age, if the mother is a good observer, the diagnosis can usually be made.

As with adults, children may suffer from all types of headache but the most common are those associated with an infectious illness, migraine or tension headaches. There are other less common types, which include headaches following head injury, headaches associated with dizziness, episodic vertigo, and, more rarely, cerebral tumours. These groups nearly all have other symptoms and signs so that they can be differentiated from the benign recurring headaches such as migraine.

MIGRAINE

As in adults, there is no diagnostic test or marker for migraine in children, so diagnosis depends entirely on the history and examination. One of the definitions of migraine in children is that it is a disorder in which there are recurrent paroxysmal headaches, between which there are symptom-free intervals, occurring in an otherwise healthy child and for which no other cause can be found. This is probably as good a definition as can be made.

Migraine is commoner in women than in men but in children before puberty the incidence is approximately 2.5 per cent in both boys and girls.

However, by the age of 11 there is an increasing predominance of girls which becomes even more marked in the 13 to 15 age group.

Migraine may begin at a very early age. In one group studied who had migraine at the age of seven, the average age of onset was 4.8 years.

Clinical features

Migraine in children does not differ very much from that in adults but the attacks are shorter, often lasting only one to four hours. Gastro-intestinal symptoms, including nausea, vomiting and abdominal pain, are much more prominent.

Children who develop migraine tend to be more likely to have suffered from recurrent abdominal pain and to have had a greater important part in migraine in children than it does in adults. Some children have attacks of unexplained abdominal pain, pallor, lethargy, nausea and vomiting, but careful questioning can usually reveal a headache.

These children who, in their early lives, do not complain of headaches, do so in otherwise similar attacks later on. A few children have classical migraine,

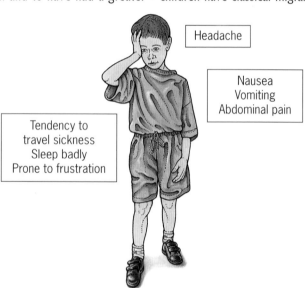

Headache

Nausea
Vomiting
Abdominal pain

Tendency to
travel sickness
Sleep badly
Prone to frustration

Clinical features of headache in children.

tendency to be travel sick than children who do not develop mi-graine. They are also more likely to sleep badly and may be more fearful, less physically strong, and more prone to frustration. Head-ache seems to play a rather less with an aura, but the incidence of this is less than in adults.

Other varieties of migraine

In common with adults, unusual migraine variants such as hemi-plegic migraine, ophthalmoplegic migraine, and migraine with dizziness and vertigo sometimes occur but are relatively rare.

Trigger factors

The trigger factors in children are mainly stress of one kind or another. These include exercise, bright lights, noise, lack of sleep, lack of food – mainly missing breakfast, cold and excitement, e.g. an approaching birthday party. These are essentially the same triggers as those for adults.

Treatment

With children, as with adults, the best treatment is to avoid the attacks by reducing the trigger factors. Meals should be regular. They must have a proper breakfast before going to school and, if possible, a proper lunch – not a snack of crisps and chocolate. Many parents fear that if their child has headaches they must be due to something serious such as a brain tumour. This is very rarely the case but if there is any doubt the child should be referred to a neurologist who will, if necessary, do full investigations.

When drug treatment is needed, the least toxic drugs should be given. In practice this means paracetamol. If sickness is a problem your doctor may prescribe an anti-nauseant such as metoclopramide or domperidone. If these are given, the doctor should warn the parents that the child may develop jerky movements. These symptoms, although not of any long-term consequence, can be disturbing so the drug should not be taken again. In the United Kingdom, aspirin is not recommended for children under the age of 12 because of the possibility that they might develop an illness known as Reye's syndrome which affects the liver and kidneys.

If adequate attack therapy is used, it is hardly ever necessary to give daily drugs to prevent attacks, and these should never be given unless the headaches are really disabling. Many parents are worried that their children may develop headaches at the times of their examinations. It is very rare for this to happen as the headaches, if they occur, nearly always do so when the exams are over.

TENSION AND MUSCLE CONTRACTION HEADACHE

Tension and muscle contraction headaches may occur in children and are relatively frequent in adolescents. These headaches may occur nearly every day. They have no specific duration – they may last for under an hour or all day.

Tension headaches differ from migraine attacks in that there are no prodromal symptoms or aura, and although sometimes the child may feel sick, he or she hardly ever vomits. As in migraine there are no abnormal physical signs and the diagnosis can only be made after taking a careful history. If possible, the child should be seen alone first, then with the parents.

Finally, the parents should be seen on their own. This is because it is the child who has the headache, and who is the only one who knows how bad the headache is and what it feels like. The parents can say how it interrupts the child's life, how often it occurs, and what tends to bring it on.

Treatment

If tension headache is the diagnosis, it must be remembered that these headaches are unlikely to respond to the drugs used in migraine although, in a few cases, paracetamol or aspirin may be helpful. The important thing is to find the cause and very often this is family friction of one kind or another. It may be that the child is using the headaches to avoid something unpleasant – the simplest of these is a wish to avoid going to school. If this is the case the reason for the dislike of school should be identified. The child may be being bullied at school, and the parents should discuss the problem with the teacher.

In other cases the child may be reacting to parental disharmony and be using the headaches either to exploit the situation or as an expression of unhappiness.

There is another small group in which the child complains of headache when the real problem is something quite different. When this is the case, the child and the family may need further medical or psychological help.

KEY POINTS

✓ Migraine may begin at a very early age.

✓ Attacks are much shorter than in adults, but abdominal pain, nausea and vomiting are more common.

✓ Lack of food is one of the trigger factors for migraine in children. They should be encouraged to eat regular meals.

✓ Tension headache in children may be caused by family friction or school phobia.

Drug treatment of migraine

Drugs are usually necessary to treat an attack but it is important not to rely on medication alone. Self-help is the most important factor in the overall management; advice on how migraine can be prevented by identifying and avoiding triggers is given on page 22.

Patients often become disillusioned because the drugs do not cure migraine. There is no cure, but drug and non-drug treatments do help to reduce the frequency and severity of attacks. The pattern of migraine changes over the years and there may be episodes of frequent attacks followed by several months or years of freedom. This means that your need for treatment may change accordingly.

Treatment of migraine falls into two main categories: acute and prophylactic (preventive). All drugs have side effects (including herbal and homoeopathic treatments) but these are usually minimal if the drugs are taken exactly as they are prescribed.

If you are given tablets to take for the acute treatment of an attack, do not take them every day to try to prevent the attacks. This can lead to problems of over-use and, in some cases, can aggravate headaches.

ACUTE TREATMENT

Drugs that you can take only when you have an attack of migraine are called acute treatments. These include painkillers bought from the pharmacy or supermarket as well as more specific treatments for migraine, which are available on prescription.

Over-the-counter drugs

Drugs from the pharmacy contain the painkiller aspirin, paracetamol or ibuprofen. Sometimes these are combined with other drugs such as codeine (a mild opiate drug) to make them more powerful or antihistamines, which help reduce nausea. Some tablets are more specifically designed for migraine. The pharmacist can advise you about these and how to take them safely. There is little difference between them so it is a matter of personal preference which you choose.

For maximum effect, take the tablets as early in the attack as possible but never take more than the maximum dose indicated. If none of them is effective or you need more than the recommended dose, you should see your doctor. If you are taking acute treatments for headache regularly on more than two or three days each week, it is possible that the treatment is making the headaches worse.

Prescription drugs

If simple painkillers are not effective, your GP may prescribe a basic anti-sickness drug, such as domperidone or metoclopramide, that also helps your usual painkillers to be absorbed into the bloodstream more effectively. Several prescription-only painkillers are used in migraine, especially when the neck and shoulder muscles are tender during attacks. These are called non-steroidal anti-inflammatory drugs (NSAIDs) and include diclofenac, naproxen and tolfenamic acid. Some drugs are available as suppositories, which are particularly useful if vomiting makes you unable to take tablets.

Drugs specific to the treatment of migraine do not act as painkillers but are thought to reduce the pain of a migraine headache by narrowing the swollen blood vessels and reversing the chemical changes in the brain that occur in migraine. One of these, ergotamine, has been used for over 70 years. The other, sumatriptan, is a new drug developed specifically for migraine. Both these drugs can be very effective but are necessary for only a minority of patients. Most sufferers can control their attacks with more simple medication, provided they are taken correctly and in sufficient time.

Ergotamine (Cafergot, Migril, Lingraine) is usually prescribed for patients in whom simple analgesics are ineffective. It is a vasoconstrictor, that is, it constricts blood vessels. It is available as tablets (some of which dissolve under the tongue) and suppositories. An inhaler, similar to the type used by asthmatics, can also be prescribed and is particularly useful for patients who feel too unwell to take tablets.

Ergotamine can aggravate nausea and vomiting, particularly if the dose is too high. This can be counteracted by taking an anti-sickness drug at the same time as you take the ergotamine. Dizziness and muscle cramps are other typical side effects. If you experience any of these symptoms, try taking a smaller dose, for example, half a tablet or half a suppository. To halve suppositories, cut the suppository down the long axis using a hot knife.

To gain maximum effect from ergotamine, take it as soon as the headache starts. The recommended dosage should not be exceeded because of the risk of ergotism or ergotamine-induced headaches. Ergotamine should not be taken by anyone with ischaemic heart disease or hypertension, as it can aggravate these conditions.

Dihydroergotamine is reported to be as effective as ergotamine with a low incidence of recurrence of migraine symptoms. Its advantage over ergotamine is that has similar, although fewer, unwanted effects. In the UK, it is available only as a nasal spray, which can have bad taste and cause local nasal symptoms such as rhinitis, stuffy nose and flushing. On the positive side, the nasal spray works quickly with effects some times seen within 15 minutes. The recommended dose is one spray in each nostril (that is, a total of two doses) at the onset of an attack. An additional one to two doses can be repeated after a minimum of 15 minutes if the first dose has not been effective. As for ergotamine, it should not be used by anyone with ischaemic heart disease or hypertension, or by anyone taking beta-blockers.

Triptans

There are four triptans currently available: naratriptan (Naramig), rizatriptan (Maxalt), sumatriptan (Imigran) and zolmitriptan (Zomig). These drugs attach to specific parts of the brain that respond to serotonin. They are thought to treat migraine by constricting only those blood vessels that become swollen during an attack, unlike ergotamine, which constricts blood vessels all over the body. Although this constricting action is localized in otherwise healthy migraine sufferers (migraineurs), certain people should not take triptans. These include people who have ischaemic heart disease or uncontrolled hypertension (high blood pressure). Anyone at potential risk of heart disease, such as someone with a close family relative who had a stroke or heart attack at an early age, smokers and people with diabetes, should be carefully checked by their doctor before taking a triptan. Typical side effects include nausea, dizziness, fatigue and feelings of heaviness in any part of the body. Recurrence of headache is another problem – the migraine attack is effectively treated but symptoms return later the same day or the following morning. This can usually be resolved by a further dose of a triptan, but can occasionally occur repeatedly over several days. Although studies suggest that triptans are effective when taken at any stage of a migraine, they are probably most effective if taken at the start of the headache. There appears to be little benefit from taking a triptan at the start of the aura of classical migraine, so it is best to wait and take the triptan when the headache develops. None of the triptans should be taken at the same time as ergotamine or other triptans.

Sumatriptan was the first triptan to be developed and it is avail-able as tablets, a self-administered injection and a nasal spray. Suma-triptan should not be taken with certain antidepressants and should be avoided by patients with a sensitivity to sulphonamides.

Naratriptan is available only as a tablet. A second dose should be used only if the migraine has responded to the first dose, but symptoms return. Naratriptan is slower to act than

PREVENTION OF MIGRAINE ATTACKS

Amitriptyline: not licensed for migraine but useful if depression is a feature
Dose: initially 10 mg each night, increasing to 75 mg if necessary
Possible side effects: dry mouth and sedation, particularly in the first two weeks

Beta-blockers: metoprolol, nadolol, propranolol and timolol can help, especially if patients are anxious or under stress. Atenolol, although not licensed for migraine, is also used
Dose: propranolol: start with 10 mg three times a day increasing after two weeks if necessary
Possible side effects: fatigue, sleep disturbance and cold extremities

Clonidine: may help women with migraine and menopausal hot flushes. Dose: 25 to 50 µg three times daily. Possible side effects: sedation, dry mouth, dizziness, depression

Cyproheptadine: an antihistamine
Dose: initially 4 mg each night
Possible side effects: dizziness and sedation

Methysergide: a derivative of ergot. Should only be administered under hospital supervision

Pizotifen: has antihistamine, antiserotonin and antidepressant properties
Dose: initially 0.5 mg each night
Possible side effects: sedation and appetite stimulation leading to increase in weight

Sodium valproate: has anti-epileptic properties
Dose: initially 200–250 mg twice daily increasing to 400–500 mg twice daily if necessary
Possible side effects: nausea, gastrointestinal disturbance, hair loss, tremor

sumatriptan but has fewer side effects. It should be avoided by those either with sensitivity to sulphonamides or usingmethysergide for preventive treatment.

Rizatriptan is available as a tablet and as a peppermint-flavoured wafer that dissolves in the mouth. This wafer is useful when nausea and vomiting are a problem, but the effect is not as rapid as a tablet. A second dose should be used only if migraine symptoms return after the initial response. A lower dose should be used by patients taking propranolol. Rizatriptan should be avoided by patients taking certain antidepressants.

Zolmitriptan is available only as a tablet. It has the advantage over other triptans that a second dose can be taken when the first dose is ineffective. A lower dose of zolmitriptan should be used by patients taking monoamine oxidase inhibitors for migraine prevention or for depression. Its use should be avoided by patients with certain heart rhythm defects such as the Wolff–Parkinson–White syndrome.

PREVENTIVE TREATMENT

If you have frequent migraines which interfere with your work or social life, your doctor may suggest that you take a course of tablets which you take every day to prevent the attacks.

These prophylactic drugs help to break the cycle so that the attacks may remain under control even when the course of treatment is complete. Prophylactic treatment is not an alternative to treating an attack so take your usual medication for any attacks that do occur.

There are many different drug treatments available but few of them are specifically designed for migraine. Do not be surprised if your doctor suggests that you take the tablets which are normally prescribed for the treatment of high blood pressure or depression. Studies show that several of these drugs are effective in the treatment of migraine, even if the person does not have high blood pressure and is not depressed.

Ask your doctor what side effects you might expect. These are usually minimal and most people tolerate them if the migraines are relieved.

Give the treatment time to take effect as too often people stop taking the tablets before they have had a chance to work. After three or four weeks you should notice an improvement. Otherwise, return to your doctor. It may be that a small adjustment in the dosage is all that is necessary, or your doctor might recommend a different treatment. If you are unhappy about taking tablets daily, tell your doctor. It is better to discuss alternatives than to go away with a prescription that you are not going to use.

Beta-blockers (for example, metoprolol, nadolol, propranolol, timolol) are useful if stress is a trigger factor or if you have high blood pressure, but should not be used in combination with ergotamine. Side effects include a lower tolerance to exercise, weight gain, fatigue, sleep disturbance and cold extremities.

Beta-blockers should not be taken by people with diabetes or asthma.

Antidepressants (for example, amitriptyline) are particularly helpful if sleep is disturbed, or migraine attacks are present on waking in the morning. Usually, a low dose is prescribed, to be taken at night. Side effects may include a dry mouth, blurred vision, constipation and sedation. These are most apparent in the first two weeks and then wear off as the drug starts to take effect.

For these reasons it is necessary to persevere with treatment for at least three weeks before assessing any side effects/benefits. Antidepressants should not be taken by patients with heart problems, epilepsy or glaucoma.

Pizotifen is a drug specifically used for the prevention of migraine. It can increase appetite, so you need to watch your diet to prevent weight gain. Sedation is another common problem, usually counteracted by taking the drug at night.

Sodium valproate is a drug more commonly used to prevent epileptic fits but which has also been shown to be an effective migraine prophylactic. Although most migraineurs tolerate the drug with few problems, it can occasionally cause some nausea, gastric upsets, hair loss, tremor and bruising. It cannot be taken by anyone who has liver problems, so liver function tests should be performed before treatment is started. It should not be taken by pregnant women.

Clonidine is an old drug used for the management of hypertension, which has shown limited efficacy for migraine prevention. It may have a particular place in the management of menopausal women with migraine and hot flushes who do not wish to take hormone replacement therapy. It should not be taken by women with a history of severe depression, because it can aggravate this.

OTHER VARIETIES OF MIGRAINE AND CLUSTER HEADACHE

The treatment of less common varieties of migraine is the same as that for classical or common migraine. Cluster headache is more difficult to treat than migraine because the pain is so severe and because each attack lasts for a relatively short time – too short for the usual painkillers to be effective; 100 per cent oxygen at the rate of seven litres per minute relieves the symptoms in about 80 per cent of attacks. More recently sumatriptan given by injection under the skin has been shown to be effective for 70 per cent of attacks. Ergotamine tartrate in doses of one milligram twice a day during the cluster may help.

Other preventive treatments are prednisone and lithium. All these treatments are available on prescription from your doctor.

Calcium channel blockers are not licensed for the treatment of migraine in the United Kingdom, although they are widely used in other countries.

Non-steroidal anti-inflammatory drugs (NSAIDs) are not usually used for the prevention of migraine, although they may occasionally be prescribed for 'menstrual' migraines. A course of NSAIDs may be recommended for patients with drug misuse headache.

KEY POINTS

✓ Drug treatment of migraine falls into two main categories – acute and preventive

✓ Acute treatment drugs should be taken as early in the attack as possible

✓ Preventive treatment drugs may take three or four weeks to have an effect

✓ Cluster headache may be treated with 100 per cent oxygen

Non-drug treatment

Nearly 70 per cent of migraine sufferers have tried alternative medical treatment at some time. Many of these help to reduce the effects of triggers, especially neck and back problems.

Most of the following treatments are unavailable on the NHS, with the exception of physiotherapy and homoeopathy. The cost can vary considerably so it is worth finding out prices before you make an appointment.

PHYSIOTHERAPY

Chartered physiotherapists normally work in conjunction with the medical profession. Look for the letters SRP or MCSP as these physiotherapists have had a three to four year initial course of training. Some physiotherapists are qualified in acupuncture, electrotherapy, and manual therapy, in addition to giving lifestyle training and advice.

NON-DRUG APPROACHES TO MIGRAINE

- Physiotherapy
- Osteopathy and chiropractic treatment
- Acupuncture
- Homoeopathy
- Yoga
- Counselling and psychotherapy
- Massage
- Alexander technique
- Herbal remedies

OSTEOPATHY AND CHIROPRACTIC

Osteopaths and chiropractors treat problems relating to bones. Chiropractors deal more specifically with disturbances of the function of the spine and its related muscles.

Chiropractors registered with the British Chiropractic Association have undertaken a four-year training course. Look for the letters MBCA, MCA or MIPC.

Similarly, registered osteopaths are entitled to use the letters GCRO or GOsC. Doctors who are osteopaths have the letters MLCON.

HERBAL REMEDIES

Studies have shown that the herb feverfew can prevent attacks of migraine. Its Latin name is *Tanacetum parthenium* and it belongs to the daisy family. Feverfew is equally effective taken as fresh leaves or tablets. A daily dose of up to four leaves or 200 milligrams is usually sufficient but no noticeable benefit may be apparent for the first six weeks. It is a drug, so there may be side effects, including mouth ulcers and stomach pain, or occasionally swollen lips. Pregnant or breast-feeding women should not take it.

Ginger and peppermint in any form can help reduce the feelings of nausea and help digestion.

Lavender oil rubbed on to the temples is another soothing remedy.

Many people with migraine have said that, when they take St John's wort, their migraine improves. To date, there are no studies to confirm these reports. The Committee on Safety of Medicines recently issued a statement advising patients taking triptans (Imigran, Maxalt, Naramig or Zomig), or a particular type of antidepressant known as SSRIs (for example, Prozac), sometimes used in migraine, to stop taking St John's wort. This is because the combination may increase the level of serotonin in the body, increasing the likelihood of side effects, including headache. The Committee on Safety of Medicines recommend that you should stop St John's wort and continue taking triptans, as prescribed, and mention this to your doctor at your next routine visit. Your other option is to continue St John's wort, in which case you should make an early appointment with your doctor to discuss your prescribed medication.

Qualified herbalists use the letters MNIMH, FNIMH, FRH or IMH.

ACUPUNCTURE

No one knows exactly how acupuncture works in preventing attacks of migraine but some sufferers find it very helpful. Pres-sing on tender points during an attack (acupressure) can also give relief.

You can find your acupressure points by gently pressing the muscles in the temples or down the back of your neck and shoulder. When you feel a tender point, press gently. Qualified acupuncturists use the letters MBAcA, FBAcA, LicAc, BAc or DrAc.

HOMOEOPATHY

The principle of homoeopathy is to treat like with like. Patients are prescribed minute amounts of substances that can imitate the symptoms of the illness. The substances recommended depend on the precise symptoms of each individual so two people with similar problems may be given different treatments. Homoeopathic treatments should only be taken on the advice of a qualified practitioner.

There are several NHS homoeopathic hospitals in the UK so discuss the possibility of a referral with your doctor if you feel it would be appropriate.

YOGA

Yoga stretches the muscles, relieves stress, helps breathing and eases tension.

Teach-yourself sound and video tapes are available from most major bookshops.

COUNSELLING AND PSYCHOTHERAPY

Everyone has problems in life but not everyone is able to deal with them. Psychotherapy can help you to identify these stresses and find ways of coming to terms with them. As stress and anxiety can trigger migraine attacks, some people may find this type of treatment beneficial.

MASSAGE

As a means of reducing tension in the muscles and providing an indulgent method of relaxation, massage can be very helpful. If performed regularly, massage can help minimize the headache result-ing from stress.

Some find massage combined with aromatic oils (aromatherapy) particularly beneficial as oils can be used to ease specific problems including poor sleep or sinus pain.

ALEXANDER TECHNIQUE

This technique was introduced by F.M. Alexander, who felt that bad posture could cause pain and illness. The emphasis is on un-learning bad habits of movement and correcting the relationship between the head and neck and the rest of the body. Such treatment may be of specific help to headache sufferers with stiff and tender neck muscles.

KEY POINTS

✓ Nearly 70 per cent of migraine sufferers have tried alternative medical treatment at some stage.

✓ Methods include the physical (physiotherapy, osteopathy and chiropractic, acupuncture, yoga, massage and Alexander technique) as well as homoeopathy, counselling and psychotherapy, and herbal remedies.

✓ Many of these are only available on a private basis.

Other types of headache

TENSION HEADACHE

Tension headache has been defined as an ache or sensation of tightness, pressure or constriction, widely varied in intensity, frequency and duration. When asked, the sufferer says it never goes and it occurs every day. Tension headache affects the whole head and, in the chronic form, it is present on waking and lasts all day.

There is a feeling of heaviness in the head or the pain may be described as a tight band around the head. Some people describe sudden jabs of pain in one area, superimposed on a general background of discomfort.

The headache may be throbbing in the early morning and develop into a dull ache during the day. In milder cases the headaches only occur during or after recognizable stress such as preparing for a dinner party or getting ready to go on holiday. In more severe cases the headaches may come on in anticipation of some unpleasant situation.

Tension headache, unlike migraine, is not associated with disturbance of sight but sufferers may have a dislike of strong light.

Sometimes they find it difficult to concentrate and they may be anxious or depressed, with the headaches made worse by any added anxieties. Patients often show signs of muscle contraction – their jaws are tense, their hands clenched, and they may drum restlessly with their fingers.

Treatment of tension headaches

If there is underlying anxiety or depression this should be treated. Patients with this type of headache should avoid taking large quantities of painkilling drugs, as taking these may lead to further problems.

Mild sedatives or tranquillizers prescribed by your family doctor are often helpful and cut down the incidence and severity of the headache but they should only be taken for a short time because of the dangers of habituation.

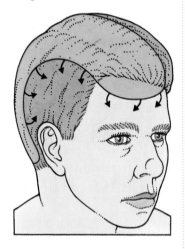

Distribution of pain in tension headache.

Reassurance is an important part of the treatment. If you are worried that the pain, which may be severe and distressing, is due to a brain tumour or other serious conditions, your doctor, after taking a history and examining you, will be able to remove your fears.

The doctor will probably also make it clear that it is improbable that you will be cured of your headache but, with treatment, the number and severity of the attacks will diminish.

This gives you control over your headaches rather than the headaches controlling you.

HEADACHE CAUSED BY EYE STRAIN

Weakness of one or more of the eye muscles

Eye muscle weakness or errors in the focusing power of the eye may occasionally cause headaches. The headache develops and increases in severity with the use of the eyes and may occur after reading, using a VDU or other prolonged close work.

There is usually discomfort and a feeling of heaviness around the eyes. The pain starts over and around the eyes, gradually increases in severity, and radiates to the forehead and temples. Sometimes there is a blurring of vision. Correction of the eye trouble by wearing appropriate spectacles improves this type of headache.

Imbalance of the eye muscles

Excessive or sustained muscle contraction in an effort to maintain normal binocular vision is another cause of headaches. A common cause is the failure of the eyes to converge and again the headache develops while reading, sewing or similar use of the eyes.

Headaches are unlikely to be caused by eye strain unless there is faulty vision or imbalance of the eye muscles so anyone who is worried about their eyes should be professionally examined and wear spectacles if they are prescribed.

DRUG MISUSE HEADACHE

Over the past few years it has become increasingly clear that too many drugs are bad for you. This is particularly so in the case of simple painkillers. Anyone who is regularly taking more that 30 painkillers a month is likely to suffer from daily headaches. These painkillers are the ones that can be bought over the counter not only from pharmacists but also from supermarkets, corner shops, etc. Most of them contain paracetamol or aspirin in a variety of forms and under many different names. If you are taking tablets daily, check what is in them. Very often on the box or package it says not to take more than six or eight per day. What it does not say is that you should not take more than 30 per month – this means a total of all tablets containing painkillers.

If you do take a lot of tablets they will not help and may be the cause of the daily headaches. The only way to make the headaches better is to stop taking the tablets.

If this is explained by their doctor, most people will accept that they are in fact poisoning themselves and are prepared to give up their tablets, especially if it is pointed out to them that, unless they do so, their headaches will continue and remain resistant to other treatments.

Other drugs used in the treatment of migraine, such as ergotamine tartrate, if taken in excess, will cause daily headaches and it cannot be emphasized too strongly that taking more than the prescribed amount of any drug can be dangerous.

SINUSITIS

In acute sinusitis the patient has a generalized headache and fever, with pain localized to the affected sinus. The pain is made worse by jolting or sudden movements, and by bending over. There may be tenderness over the affected sinus and sometimes slight swelling of the lower eyelid. Sinusitis is usually treated with antibiotics and decongestants.

Vague discomfort on the forehead, between the eyes, and across the nose, is often thought to be due to chronic sinusitis but in most cases there is no evidence of sinus infection. If in doubt, you should ask your doctor to refer you to an ear, nose and throat specialist.

HEADACHE FROM HIGH BLOOD PRESSURE

A moderately high blood pressure is quite common and does not cause headache. Blood pressure which is really high may do so, and

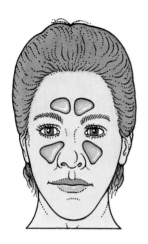
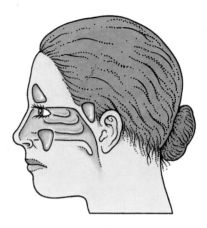

Headache and tenderness over the affected sinus may be symptoms of acute sinusitis.

in these patients reducing the pressure will probably relieve the headache. Headaches caused by high blood pressure are usually at the back of the head, present on waking, and are pulsating or throbbing in nature. Many people who have been told that they have high blood pressure are worried about this, and often these headaches improve with reas-surance, rest and sufficient sleep. In any case, the treatment of high blood pressure is now very effective.

HEAD INJURY

Most people complain of headache after a head injury where the injury is relatively mild and the patient has not lost consciousness.

The headache usually wears off after a few hours or days. However mild the injury, it is as well to rest, pre-ferably lying flat in bed, until the headache has gone. Simple pain-killers such as aspirin and parace-tamol can be used.

When the injury is more severe and the patient has been uncon-scious, even for a short time, it is important to consult the doctor. The patient may be admitted to hospital overnight, as occasionally bleeding inside the head may occur and cause further symptoms.

Slowing of the pulse, drow-siness and unconsciousness are signs of bleeding in the head. This bleeding may raise the intracranial pressure, which requires surgical treatment.

HEADACHE CAUSED BY THE NECK

Most of the population over the age of 40 have changes of cervical spondylosis (immobility of the neck region) in their spine and these can be seen on X-ray. In most people these do not cause any symptoms but, occasionally, changes in the upper part of the cervical spine may cause pain in the back of the neck which extends up the back of the head.

The commonest neck injury is known as whiplash which typically follows a car crash. In this type of accident the neck is stretched back and forth beyond its normal range.

Following the injury there is widespread soreness in the neck which is followed, in hours or days, by more generalized neck and head pains which are made worse by movement. The head pain, in the early stages, is felt as a continuation of the neck pain and spreads upwards from the back of the head to the forehead and may be one-sided or overall. The pain is usually described as dull or heavy, and is made worse by sudden neck movements.

In most people the pain goes away in a few days or weeks but sometimes it persists and the full whiplash syndrome develops. The resulting headache is described as a severe widespread pain which is worst first thing in the morning, during mental or physical exertion, and with certain neck movements. Other neck movements and postures may ease the pain.

The associated symptoms include vague dizziness, noises in the ears, discomfort in the throat, impaired memory and concentration, and fatigue. On examination there is slight tenderness in the muscles of the neck and the back of the head, and the head is held stiffly. The treatment comprises rest, painkillers, a cervical collar and physiotherapy. The collar should only be worn until the pain diminishes because complete recovery will not take place until the neck muscles recover their strength.

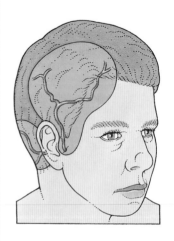

Distribution of pain in temporal arteritis.

TEMPORAL ARTERITIS

Temporal arteritis (or inflammation of the arteries of the head) affects people over the age of 50, particularly women. It usually starts with pain over the affected scalp vessels (often those in the temples). The arteries become thickened, cease to pulsate, are tender when touched, and the skin over the artery becomes red. Most patients complain of headache, the pain being on one or both sides and worse over the affected vessels. Sometimes chewing causes pain in the muscles of the jaw.

The disorder may affect blood vessels inside the head as well as the temporal artery, particularly the artery that supplies the eye. If this happens, impairment of vision or blindness may result so if you are over 50 and develop a severe headache and do not feel well, go and see your doctor at once. Steroids rapidly ease the pain, and temporal arteritis responds well to treatment but you may have to continue treatment for a long time.

BRAIN TUMOURS

Many people with constant or recurring headache are worried because they think the pain may be caused by a brain tumour. This is very unlikely because brain tumours are relatively rare and headaches, as the sole symptom, are hardly ever due to a tumour. If your headache is associated with weakness or unpleasant sensations in the arm or leg, you should consult your family doctor, who can refer you to a specialist.

KEY POINTS

✓ Other types of headache include tension headache, and headaches caused by drug misuse, eye strain, sinusitis, high blood pressure, whiplash injury, temporal arteritis and brain tumours.

✓ Taking more than the prescribed amount of any drug is dangerous.

✓ Headaches are hardly ever the only symptom of a tumour.

The future

In spite of the fact that migraine has been recognized for more than 3000 years, there were minimal advances in our understanding of its mechanisms until this century.

The earliest known reference to migraine is recorded on a papyrus written in 1200 BC, found in the tomb of Thebes. It records a magic spell said to be effective against a type of headache known as half temple.

Treatments have ranged from prayers and incantations, to the positively dangerous art of trepanation, in an attempt to expel the demons thought to be responsible for the affliction. Trepanation is the removal of a segment of bone from the skull; skulls dating from 7000 BC show signs of trepanation although it is not known if this was a specific treatment for headache. However, there is evidence that trepanation was performed as a treatment for intractable migraine in seventeenth century France.

Other historical treatments are more likely to have had some effect. One remedy dating from Egyptian times was to bind a clay crocodile around the head of the sufferer using a strip of linen on which were written the names of the gods. The resulting pressure on the scalp might have eased the pain.

GOALS IN DRUG RESEARCH

At present, the pharmaceutical industry is in competition to create new drugs that are more effective and safer than their predecessors. Although serotonin is currently the focus of attention, it is only one of numerous chemical messengers within the human body and does not act in isolation. The fact that many substances used in the treatment of migraine affect serotonin mechanisms is insufficient evidence to implicate serotonin as the cause. There may be other chemicals, some not yet identified, which play a more significant role.

Further research is vital as a great deal about migraine remains a mystery – proof for many of the theories remains elusive and many questions are unanswered. Many factors other than headache need to be accounted for. For example, no one knows how, or why, triggers ranging from strong smells to drinking alcohol trigger an attack, or why some people experience a warning aura, or suffer nausea and vomiting, all of which make migraine so different from a simple headache.

Ideally, understanding the mechanism of an attack will help doctors develop ways to manage migraine with minimal use of drugs.

PROBING THE GENETIC LINK

The argument that migraine is an inherited condition is not new but in a condition as common as migraine it is likely that each patient will be aware of at least one other family member who experiences attacks, without there being a genetic link. One problem in genetic research is the necessity of correct diagnosis. For example, if all the members of a family affected by migraine cannot be effectively identified, perhaps because one or two of them have infrequent attacks which they do not recognize as migraine, then this will obviously affect the outcome of any study. A further problem is that migraine appears to result from a complex combination of internal and external factors which interact, and is not the result of one factor alone.

Even with these limitations, doctors are keen to find out if there is a true genetic basis for migraine. It has long been thought that the genetic link is the inheritance of a migraine threshold – the susceptibility to migraine. Recent advances in genetics have made it easier to isolate specific genes, and the identification of a gene for migraine is theoretically possible.

A TEST FOR MIGRAINE

Currently, there are no investigations available that can confirm the diagnosis of migraine: the diagnosis rests solely on the story related by the patient to the doctor, in the absence of other symptoms or physical findings. Tests are only necessary if there is any uncertainty about the diagnosis and other causes of headache need to be excluded.

The history of the attacks and physical examination are usually sufficient for most doctors to make a confident diagnosis but it may not be so easy for someone with limited experience. To enable a more accurate evaluation, researchers are trying to devise a test that could positively identify all patients with migraine without producing any false results.

Maybe when a greater understanding of the mechanism of the attack is reached, or if a specific gene is identified, it will be possible to produce a test.

CHANGING ATTITUDES TO MIGRAINE

Perhaps the most significant advance has been in the changing attitudes towards migraine. It is now recognized as an organic condition with measurable biochemical changes – a far cry from the belief that it was a neurotic condition and all in the mind.

The increased amount of research has also raised the profile of migraine, leading sufferers to realize that they are not alone.

Although a cure for migraine remains elusive, there are several treatments, both drug and non-drug, available to help people cope with attacks.

We have come a long way since prayer or drilling holes in the skull were the only treatments on offer. But the main answer to migraine lies with the patients. There is a great deal that migraine sufferers can do to help themselves, verified by the success of the Migraine Action Association, a self-help group.

To advance our knowledge further, it would be of great value to identify accurately the real extent of migraine in the population. Much of this would depend on raising the profile of migraine further, helping people to realize that their headaches may be migraine, teaching them how to deal with the attacks, and expelling any remaining myths.

KEY POINTS

✓ The pharmaceutical industry is continually trying to find new drugs that will be more effective than their predecessors.

✓ Identification of a gene for migraine is theoretically possible.

✓ Researchers are trying to devise a test that could positively identify all patients with migraine without producing false results.

Questions & answers

● Having had my first migraine at the age of 25 can I expect to suffer from it for the rest of my life?

The answer to this is probably no but it varies considerably from person to person. Migraine is essentially a disorder of the young, the first headache usually occurring before the age of 20. One survey showed that the average age of those attending a migraine clinic was 38. Most people find that their headaches diminish as they reach middle age and may disappear completely. In a small minority, they may persist until later life.

The reason why most patients' headaches improve in middle life is not known. Various theories have been put forward. One is that by middle age life becomes less stressful and therefore headaches due to stress are less likely. Another is that in women after the menopause, the hormonal pattern becomes more regular and the withdrawal of oestrogen which sometimes precipitates a headache no longer occurs. Yet another theory is that as one grows older the blood vessels do not react so readily to circulatory substances and therefore are less liable to dilate or constrict.

● Can lying out in the sun for long periods cause headache?

Lying out in the sun may cause headache if the individual becomes sunburnt, although some people are sensitive to even short exposure to the sun. The more severe condition, hyperthermia, occurs when the exposure is longer and is accompanied by dehydration. The symptoms of this are a high temperature and very severe headache. If you are in a hot country it is essential to take adequate amounts of fluid and salt.

● Does artificial lighting, particularly the fluorescent type, cause headache?

Artificial lighting as a rule is not as good as normal daylight and if the illumination is inadequate this may be the cause of headache – probably because of eye strain. Fluorescent lighting usually gives a good light but may flicker. In sensitive people this may cause headache. Where fluorescent lighting is used it is important to see that it is properly adjusted so that flickering does not occur. Recurrent flashing lights may also cause headache.

People working with VDUs sometimes complain of headaches. This is partly because they are looking at a small bright screen for long periods of time. If using a VDU it is important to relax from time to time (ideally, experts recommend users have breaks every 20 minutes) and if you feel that your neck is stiff, do some simple stretching exercises.

● I have heard that sexual intercourse can trigger headaches. Is this true?

Headaches can be linked to sexual activity. The condition has been called a number of different names: benign sex headache, benign coital headache, orgasmic or coital cephalgia, and thunderclap headache – describing the explosive nature of the attack, which can be very frightening.

Fortunately, it is rare for there to be any serious underlying cause but the condition is extremely unpleasant. A few patients experience regular attacks with intercourse, others have several unpredictable episodes – sometimes with a gap of many years.

The pain starts as orgasm is reached and feels like a dull cramp at the back of the head. It is usually very intense for the first 5–15 minutes, following which it may disappear. Sometimes it will continue as a dull ache for up to 24 hours. Muscular spasm in the neck is the most likely cause but anyone experiencing these headaches should see their doctor to confirm the diagnosis.

Useful addresses

REGISTERED MEDICAL CHARITIES

Please enclose a stamped, addressed envelope for a reply when writing to these organizations.

City of London Migraine Clinic
22 Charterhouse Square
London EC1M 6DX
Tel: 020 7251 3322
Fax: 020 7490 2183

A medical charity that sees patients from any part of the country. A GP referral letter is required for an appointment. Patients are given emergency treatment at the start of an attack if they are existing patients.

Migraine Action Association (formerly British Migraine Association)
178a High Road
Byfleet
West Byfleet KT14 7ED
Tel: 01932 352468
Fax: 01932 351257
Email: info@migraine.org.uk
Website: www.migraine.org.uk

This charity is run by migraine sufferers for migraine sufferers. A newsletter is published every three months.

Migraine Trust
45 Great Ormond Street
London WC1N 3HZ
Tel: 020 7831 4818 (helpline and general enquiries)
Fax: 020 7831 5174
Email: migrainetrust@compuserve.com
Website: www.migrainetrust.org

A charity that promotes research and provides information for migraine sufferers.

OTHER MIGRAINE CLINICS

There are several migraine clinics in London and around the UK. For information on local clinics, contact Migraine Action Association (see above).

Princess Margaret Migraine Clinic
Charing Cross Hospital
Fulham Palace Road
London W6 8RF
Tel: 020 8846 1234
Fax: 020 8846 7715
An NHS clinic.

Index

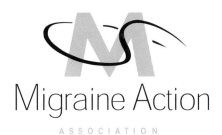

Migraine Action

ASSOCIATION

Patient Support Group formed in 1958

It has three principal aims:

- to provide support and encouragement to migraine sufferers, their families and friends
- to raise awareness of this disability and much misunderstood condition which affects approximately 10% of the population
- to encourage and support research into the causes, diagnosis and treatment of migraine.

Regular newsletter and variety of information leaflets on all aspects of migraine. Membership fee £5.00 per year.

Migraine Action Association
(formerly British Migraine Association)
178a High Road, Byfleet, West Byfleet,
Surrey KT14 7ED
Telephone: 01932 352468

Registered as a Charity Number 207783